Bath Bombs
Beginner Bath Bomb Recipes for Aromatherapy, Stress Reduction, and Better Health

Table of Contents

Copyright

Introduction

I want to thank and congratulate you for downloading the book "*Bath Bombs: Bath Bomb Recipes for Aromatherapy, Stress Reduction, and Better Health!*"

Bath time is supposed to be a time where you can relax and let go of all the tension that you feel. After all, it's a time that you can spend alone.

Because of the hustle and bustle of life, it's sometimes hard to feel like you still have time to relax and enjoy. Well, you can do so during bath time—with the help of bath bombs that are therapeutic, calming, and would make the state of your health better!

With the help of this book, you'll learn how to make the best bath bombs that will help you relax and would make you healthier and happier! Start reading this book now and make those bath bombs as soon as you can!

Once again, thank you and enjoy!

Chapter 1: Romantic and Light Bath Bombs

When you want to relax your mind and feel better, you need to set a romantic and light mood because it will help you realize that you're okay and that life is great. Well, this is easy to do during bath time, especially when you have the right bath bombs with you—and you'll learn how to make some of them in this chapter!

Hearty Bath Bombs

Grapefruit is an anti-depressant so it can definitely lighten up your mood and make you feel relaxed!

What you'll need:

Heart Molds

8 oz Mason Jars

1/2 Tbsp Jojoba Oil

1/2 cup of Citric Acid

1 cup baking soda

1/4 cup of extra fine Epsom Salt

3 drops Grapefruit Essential Oil

1 Tbsp Pink Brazilian Clay

Witch Hazel Spray

Instructions:

In a bowl, mix Epson Salt, Citric Acid and Baking Soda altogether.   This will lead to clump formation, but don't worry about that.

Sift until you see that there are no more clumps. Use a strainer to do so.
Next, add the Grapefruit Essential Oil and the Jojoba Oil then mix them together until a powdery mixture appears.

Divide the mixture into two.

Leave one of them uncolored then add the Pink Brazilian Clay into the other one. Mix until well-combined.

Next, spray some Witch Hazel on the bombs. Do it for at least 8 to 10 times then add some Jojoba Oil, too, so they would really stick together.

Press both of the mixtures into the heart molds and pack. Leave them there until they're hard enough. Doing so overnight would be good.

The next day, take them out of the molds and place them in the Mason Jars. Voila! You now have some Hearty Bath Bombs with you!

Sage and Lavender Surprise

Lavender is very calming. Take a bath at night with this bath bomb and you'll surely be able to sleep better!

What you'll need:

560 grams baking soda
250 grams citric acid
Lavender flowers
Small rose buds
Witch Hazel Spray
40 drops Green Soap Colorant
10 drops Lavender Essential Oil
10 drops Sage Essential Oil
5 grams Olive Oil
5 grams Castor Oil
6 grams Lavender Flower Powder
10 grams Bentonite Clay

Instructions:

Prepare one bowl for dry ingredients and another bowl for wet ingredients.

Mix baking soda, citric acid, lavender flower powder and bentonite clay in the first bowl then mix olive oil, lavender essential oil, sage essential oil, castor oil, and soap colorant in the other bowl.

Add the wet and dry ingredients together and

mix until well combined.
Spray Witch Hazel into the mixture gradually and continue mixing until the mixture is crumbly.

Arrange rose buds and lavender flowers on the mold then press the mixture onto them.
Wait for the mixture to dry then you can use it.
Enjoy!

Everything's coming up Roses

Roses are popular not only because they are delicate and beautiful, but also because they symbolize romance! They're soothing and can definitely put a smile on your face, too!

What you'll need:

¼ cup Rose Petals, dried
10 to 15 drops Rose Essential Oil
5 drops food coloring
½ Tbsp water
½ cup Citric Acid
2 tsp Almond Oil
1 ½ cups Baking Soda

Instructions:
In a bowl, mix rose petals with baking soda until well combined.

Mix with citric acid and food coloring.

Add almond oil and mix until moist before adding Rose Essential Oil.

Add some water if the mixture is too crumbly then make a ball out of the mixture by using your hands then press it down onto a mold. Let the mixture stay there until it is hard and dry then store in an airtight container. Take note that this one may take a few days before it totally gets hard.
Enjoy!

Jazzy Jasmine Bomb

Jasmine is a natural aphrodisiac and is also an anti-depressant so it would definitely make you feel better!

What you'll need:

1/3 cup Epsom Salt
½ cup Corn Starch
½ cup of Citric Acid
1 cup Baking Soda
Witch Hazel Spray
¼ tsp Borax
1 tsp Vitamin E Oil
¼ tsp Jasmine Essential Oil
¾ Tbsp water
2 ½ Tbsp Sweet Almond Oil

Instructions:

Combine corn starch, citric acid and baking soda in a bowl and sift.

After sifting, add Epsom Salt then set the mixture aside.

Now, it's time to mix the wet ingredients together. In a small jar, mix sweet almond oil, water, Jasmine Essential Oil, Vitamin E Oil, and Borax altogether. Put the lid of the jar on and mix the ingredients until well combined.

Mix wet and dry ingredients together and mix until crumbly. Spray some Witch Hazel if the mixture feels too dry then press the mixture onto the molds and leave them there for a couple of hours or until dry.

After a few hours, take them out of the molds and air dry them for around a week, covered with wax paper.

Once a week has passed, you can now use and enjoy your Jasmine bath bombs!

Vanilla Baby

Research has it men love the smell of Vanilla on women and Vanilla has this sweet and relaxing scent that's just perfect for everyone!

What you'll need:

1/3 cup Epsom Salt
½ cup Corn Starch
½ cup of Citric Acid
1 cup Baking Soda
Witch Hazel Spray
Liquid Food Coloring
2 ½ Tbsp Grapeseed Oil
¼ tsp Borax
1 tsp Vitamin E Oil
15 to 20 drops Vanilla Essential Oil
¾ Tbsp water

Instructions:

Combine corn starch, citric acid and baking soda in a bowl and sift.

After sifting, add Epsom Salt then set the mixture aside.

Now, it's time to mix the wet ingredients together. In a small jar, mix sweet almond oil, water, Vanilla Essential Oil, Borax, and Vitamin E Oil altogether.

Close the jar and shake until ingredients are well combined.

Mix wet and dry ingredients together and mix until crumbly. Spray some Witch Hazel if the mixture feels too dry then press the mixture onto the molds and leave them there for a couple of hours or until dry.

Take the hardened bath bombs out of the molds then cover them with wax paper. Wait for it to dry some more for about a week then use.

Chapter 2: Antioxidant Bombs

If you look good, chances are you'd also feel good about yourself. Now, when you feel good about yourself, you can expect that your health will also be in tip top shape because you won't be boggled by all these thoughts. In this chapter, you'll learn how to make bath bombs that are full of anti-oxidants that can give you radiant looking skin and a better disposition in life! Check them out.

Oh my Cherry Bomb

This bath bomb is best used before sleeping at night as cherries calm the mind and rejuvenate the body—making you feel young and healthy!

What you'll need:

9 grams Beet Root Powder
9 grams Bentonite Clay
40 drops Cherry Essential Oil
10 grams Olive Oil
14 grams Castor Oil
1, 120 grams baking soda
Witch Hazel Spray
512 grams Citric Acid

Instructions:

In a bowl, mix baking soda, citric acid, and beet root powder altogether.

Then, add some bentonite clay and mix to enhance the color of the dry mixture.
In another bowl, combine olive oil, castor oil, and Cherry Essential Oil together and mix until well combined.

Mix wet and dry ingredients together and gradually spray Witch Hazel until you see that the ingredients have formed a crumbly mixture then press half of the mixture onto the mold. Then press the other half on another mold.

Spray some Witch Hazel on both of the molds then press them together and wait for them to dry. Take out the cherry bath bombs from the molds then use and enjoy.

Blueberry Madness

Blueberries contain a lot of antioxidants that are great when it comes to making hair shiny, and letting your skin be soft and supple. Enjoy bath time even more with this great bath bomb!

What you'll need:

Witch Hazel Spray
10 grams blue fun colorant
5 grams blueberry fruit powder
40 drops Blueberry Essential Oil
18 grams Sweet Almond Oil
1, 120 grams baking soda

512 grams Citric Acid

Instructions:

In a bowl, baking soda with citric acid then add fruit powder. Mix with your hands and make sure to break any clumps apart.

Then, in another bowl, combine sweet almond oil, Blueberry Essential Oil, and soap colorant altogether. Mix until well combined.

Mix the wet ingredients with the dry ingredients and mix them with your hands until well-combined.

Spray some Witch Hazel then continue mixing until mixture turns crumbly.
Press the mixture onto the molds and wait for them to dry.

After drying, take bath bombs out of the molds and use.
Enjoy!

Fruity Peach Bomb

What you'll need:

½ cup corn starch
1 cup baking soda
1/3 cup Epsom Salt
½ cup Citric Acid
Witch Hazel Spray
Orange food coloring
1 tsp Vitamin E Oil
2 ½ Tbsp sweet almond oil
20 drops Peach Essential Oil
10 drops Peach Fragrance Oil
¾ Tbsp water

Instructions:

In a bowl, combine Epsom Salt, Citric Acid, Baking Soda, and Corn Starch altogether. Sift until you have let go of clumps.

In a bowl, mix water, sweet almond oil, Peach Essential Oil, Peach Fragrance Oil, food coloring, and Vitamin E Oil altogether.
Mix until well-combined.

Mix wet and dry ingredients together and mix until crumbly. Spray some Witch Hazel if the mixture feels too dry then press the mixture onto the molds and leave them there for a couple of hours or until dry.

Take the hardened bath bombs out of the molds then cover them with wax paper. Wait for it to dry some more for about a week then use and enjoy!

Green Tea Bath Bomb

Green Tea is not just for drinking! This anti-oxidant packed product can also be used to make a bath bomb that's soothing and relaxing. Here's how.

What you'll need:

2 cups baking soda
½ cup cornstarch
1 cup citric acid
12 drops tea tree oil
3 Tbsp Green Tea leaves
Boiling water
3 Tbsp jojoba oil
Liquid food coloring
½ cup Epsom Salt
1 Tbsp Green Tea Powder

Instructions:

Boil some water and take around a teaspoon of it and drop it over the green tea leaves so they will be hydrated. Set aside.

In a bowl, mix green tea powder, cornstarch,

baking soda, and citric acid together. Mix until well combined.

In another bowl, combine liquid food coloring, tea tree oil, jojoba oil, water, and green tea leaves altogether. Mix until well combined.
Pour wet ingredients over dry ingredients then mix them with your hands until crumbly. Add more water if it's too crumbly then press the mixture into the molds and let them dry for around 12 to 24 hours.

Use bath bombs and enjoy!

Milky Strawberry Bomb

Strawberries smell so yummy especially when you bathe with them! They can hydrate your skin and make it softer and smoother—and that's why you need this bath bomb now!

What you'll need:

Witch Hazel Spray
½ oz Strawberry Fragrance Oil
12 drops Strawberry Essential Oil
2 cups baking soda
1 cup dried Rose Petals
1 cup citric acid
Pink liquid food coloring
Bentonite Clay

Instructions:

In a bowl, mix baking soda, Bentonite Clay, and citric acid altogether.

Add Rose Petals and mix until well combined. In another bowl, mix Strawberry Essential Oil, Fragrance Oil, and liquid food coloring until well combined.

Pour wet ingredients over dry ingredients then mix with your hands until crumbly. Spray Witch Hazel gradually until you can make balls out of the mixture.

Press mixture into bath bomb molds and let them dry overnight or until 48 hours, if desired. Store in mason jars or airtight containers and use.

Chapter 3: Citrusy Bath Bombs

Citrus fruits or ingredients can definitely make you feel better inside and out. For one, they smell nice and they can clear your head, plus they can also keep you safe from common colds and flu— even in bath bomb forms! When your bathroom smells nice, chances are, your health will be a whole lot better, too!

Marjoram and Eucalyptus Mix

The great thing about this bath bomb is that it smells extremely nice—and it can clear up those nasal passages!

What you'll need:

1/3 cup Sea Salt
½ cup Corn Starch
½ cup Citric Acid
1 cup Baking Soda
Liquid Food Coloring
5 drops Ravensara Essential Oil
3 drops Strawberry Essential Oil
5 drops Eucalyptus Essential Oil
5 drops Marjoram Essential Oil
5 drops Lavender Essential Oil
Witch Hazel Spray
¾ Tbsp water
2 ½ Jojoba Oil

Instructions:

In a sifter, mix corn starch, citric acid and baking soda together. Sift until there are no more clumps then add Sea Salt and mix until well combined.

In a jar, combine jojoba oil, water, essential oils, and liquid food coloring together until well combined.

Combine wet and dry ingredients together and mix with your hands until crumbly. Spray Witch Hazel to add mist and prevent it from being too dry.

Press mixture into the molds and wait for them to dry overnight.

To harden it even more and make it more fragrant, cover in wax paper and air dry for a week after drying overnight.|

Use and enjoy!

Tea Tree Bomb

Tea Tree Oil not only relaxes the mind, it also repels insects away and can even strengthen your respiratory system—which makes this bath bomb something that you really should try!

What you'll need:

Witch Hazel Spray
10 drops Tea Tree Essential Oil
5 drops Lavender Essential Oil
2 ½ Tbsp Grapeseed Oil
Liquid food coloring
½ cup corn starch
½ cup citric acid
1 cup baking soda
1/3 cup Epsom Salt

Instructions:

Combine corn starch, citric acid and baking soda together in a sifter. Sift until there are no more clumps then add Epsom Salt and mix until well combined.

In a jar, combine essential oils, Grapeseed oil and liquid food coloring and close the lid of the jar. Shake until well combined.

Combine wet and dry ingredients together and mix with your hands until crumbly. Spray Witch

Hazel to add mist and prevent it from being too dry.

Press mixture into the molds and wait for them to dry overnight.

Take bath bombs out of the molds and cover in wax paper to air dry for a week.

Use and enjoy!

Orange Coco Bomb

Coconut Oil is very beneficial especially when it comes to strengthening the immune system and keeping the body safe from diseases. Orange also has great respiratory benefits which makes this bath bomb a really healthy one!

What you'll need:

1/3 cup sea salt
½ cup Citric Acid
1 cup baking soda
½ cup cornstarch
¼ tsp Coconut Essential Oil
½ tsp Orange Essential Oil
Witch Hazel Spray
3 Tbsp water
Liquid food coloring
2 ½ Tbsp Jojoba Oil

Instructions:

Use a sifter to combine mix corn starch, citric acid and baking soda together. Sift until there are no more clumps then add Sea Salt and mix until well combined.

In a jar, combine jojoba oil, water, essential oils, and liquid food coloring together. Place the lid on the jar and shake until ingredients are well-combined.

Combine wet and dry ingredients together and mix with your hands until crumbly. Spray Witch Hazel to add mist and prevent it from being too dry.

Press mixture into the molds and wait for them to dry overnight.

To harden it even more and make it more fragrant, cover in wax paper and air dry for a week after drying overnight.

Use and enjoy!

All Hail Lemon

Lemon may be too sour or tangy for you, but it has all these amazing health benefits—and now you can experience them through this bath bomb!

What you'll need:

1 cup baking soda
½ cup cornstarch
10 drops lemon essential oil
1/3 cup Epsom Salt
½ cup Citric Acid
Witch Hazel Spray
3 Tbsp water
Liquid food coloring
2 ½ Tbsp Grapeseed Oil

Instructions:

Combine baking soda, corn starch, and citric acid together in a sifter then sift until there are no more clumps then add Epsom Salt and mix until well combined.

In a jar, combine Grapeseed oil, water, liquid food coloring, and lemon essential oil together. Place the lid on the jar and shake until ingredients are well-combined.

Combine wet and dry ingredients together and mix with your hands until crumbly. Spray Witch Hazel to add mist and prevent it from being too dry.

Press mixture into the molds and wait for them to dry overnight.

If you want a bath bomb that's more fragrant, let it air dry, covered with wax paper for around a week.

Use and enjoy!

Lime and Ylang Ylang Bath Bomb

Well, this may sound like an unusual combination but it's something that you'd definitely love because it's relaxing and it strengthens the respiratory system. Here are some that you can try.

What you'll need:

2 ½ Tbsp Grapeseed Oil
1 cup baking soda
1/3 cup Sea Salt
½ up cornstarch
10 drops lime essential oil
10 drops Ylang Ylang Essential Oil
½ cup Citric Acid
Witch Hazel Spray
3 Tbsp water
Liquid food coloring

Instructions:

Combine baking soda, corn starch, and citric acid together in a sifter. Sift until there are no more clumps then add Sea Salt and mix until well combined.

In a jar, combine lime essential oil, Ylang Ylang Essential Oil, Grapeseed oil and liquid food coloring and close the lid of the jar. Shake until well combined.

Combine wet and dry ingredients together and mix with your hands until crumbly. Spray Witch Hazel to add mist and prevent it from being too dry.

Press mixture into the molds and wait for them to dry overnight.

Take bath bombs out of the molds and cover in wax paper to air dry for a week.

Use and enjoy!

Chapter 4: All the Happy Bombs

The bath bombs in this chapter are guaranteed to heighten your mood and make you happier! Check them out below.

Rosewood and Bergamot Surprise

The combination of these two oils might not be so usual, but once you try them, you'll realize how good they are and how they could make your mood better!

What you'll need:

10 drops Rosewood Essential Oil
10 drops Bergamot Essential oil
Witch Hazel Spray
1/3 cup Epsom Salt
3 Tbsp water
½ cup Baking Soda
½ cup Corn Starch
¼ cup Citric Acid
2 ½ Tbsp Jojoba Oil

Instructions:

In a sifter, combine baking soda, corn starch, and citric acid together. Sift until there are no more clumps then add Epsom Salt and mix until well combined.
In a jar, combine jojoba oil, Bergamot Essential

Oil, Rosewood Essential Oil and liquid food coloring and close the lid of the jar. Shake until well combined.

Combine wet and dry ingredients together and mix with your hands until crumbly. Spray Witch Hazel to add mist and prevent it from being too dry.

Press mixture into the molds and wait for them to dry overnight.

Take bath bombs out of the molds and cover in wax paper to air dry for a week.

Use and enjoy!

Cotton Candy Bomb

Who doesn't like cotton candy? Well, you may not eat it a lot anymore but you can bring cotton candy back into your life with the help of this bath bomb!

What you'll need:

4 grams Neon Pink soap colorant
4 grams Neon Blue soap colorant
40 drops Cotton Candy Fragrance Oil
2 grams sweet almond oil
6 grams castor oil
12 grams Bentonite Clay

596 grams Baking Soda
134 grams Cornstarch
292 grams Citric Acid

Instructions:

Put each of the colorants in separate bowls then set aside.

In one bowl, mix baking soda, citric acid, bentonite clay, and cornstarch altogether and mix until well-combined.

In another bowl, combine cotton candy fragrance oil, castor oil, and sweet almond oil altogether the mix until well-combined.

Combine wet and dry ingredients together and mix with your hands until crumbly.
Gradually spray Witch Hazel to mist the mixture.

Cut the mixture in half and combine one with the blue colorant and the other one with the pink. Mix then press each of them into the molds.

Once they're dry, spray each of them with Witch Hazel then press both of the molds together.

Once bath bombs are dry, take them out of the molds and air dry them for 2 more hours before storing in airtight containers. Enjoy!

Faith, Trust, and Fairy Dust

Feel like a fairy with this bath bomb that combines the essences of Vanilla and Jasmine!

What you'll need:

4 grams Fairy Dust Fragrance Oil
20 grams Vanilla Powder
11 grams Jasmine Flowers
1 gram Diamond Dust Mica
56 grams Citric Acid
112 grams baking soda

Instructions:

In a bowl, combine baking soda, Jasmine flowers, Citric Acid, Vanilla Powder, and Mica altogether then add fairy dust oil and mix until well-combined.
Press into bath bomb molds and wait overnight for them to dry out.
Store in mason jars then use and enjoy!

My Dose of Happiness Bomb

Made with Geranium that's sure to soothe your soul and put a smile on your face, you definitely have to try this bath bomb!

What you'll need:

5 drops Geranium Essential Oil
5 drops Bergamot Essential Oil
5 drops Peppermint Essential Oil
Witch Hazel Spray
Liquid food coloring
¾ Tbsp water
½ cup baking soda
¼ cup citric acid
2 ½ Tbsp Jojoba Oil
1/3 cup Sea Salt
½ cup cornstarch

Instructions:

In a sifter, combine baking soda, corn starch, and citric acid together. Sift until there are no more clumps then add Sea Salt and mix until well combined.

In a jar, combine jojoba oil, Geranium Essential Oil Bergamot Essential Oil, Peppermint Essential Oil and liquid food coloring and close the lid of the jar. Shake until well combined. Combine wet and dry ingredients together and mix with your hands until crumbly. Spray Witch

Hazel to add mist and prevent it from being too dry.

Press mixture into the molds and wait for them to dry overnight.

Take bath bombs out of the molds and cover in wax paper to air dry for a week.
Use and enjoy!

Chapter 5: Colorful and Special Bath Bombs

Finally, here are some bath bombs that you can make that are perfect as gifts and can be used for different seasons and occasions. They're also made with some of the most exciting ingredients—which will surely make you happy!

Rainbow Connection

Indulge in your bath with this cool combination of ingredients that will surely help you cool down!

What you'll need:

30 drops Rainbow Sherbet Fragrance Oil
105 grams Coconut Oil 76
68 grams Arrowroot Powder
228 grams baking soda
8 drops Neon Pink Colorant
8 drops Lime Green Colorant
8 drops Orange Colorant
84 grams Citric Acid
Witch Hazel Spray

Instructions:

Melt coconut oil 76 in a microwave bowl then set aside.

Then, combine baking soda, arrowroot powder, and citric acid in a bowl and mix with your hands until well combined.

Separate each of the colorants into different bowls and set aside.

Pour coconut oil 76 into the bowl with the ingredients and mix until there are no more clumps. Add Rainbow Sherbet Fragrance Oil and stir until well-combined.

Place equal amounts of the mixture to each of the colorants and mix until crumbly.

Press each of the bowls with the ingredients into the molds then wait for them to dry.

After drying, spray Witch Hazel over each of them then press them altogether.

Wait for 24 hours so they will dry properly then take them out and store in airtight containers.

Use and enjoy!

Easter Egg Bombs

Take Easter into a whole new different level with this fun bath bomb recipe! With the use of jellybeans and Peppermint, this will surely heighten up your mood and make you feel better about yourself!

What you'll need:

Easter egg Molds
30 drops Jellybeans Fragrance Oil
10 drops Peppermint Essential Oil
21 grams Olive Oil
26 grams Castor Oil
11 grams Bentonite Clay Powder
90 grams Arrowroot Powder
265 grams Baking Soda
184 grams Citric Acid
5 drops Ultramarine Violet food colorant
4 drops Neon Yellow food colorant
6 drops Neon Red food colorant
4 drops Neon Blue food colorant

Instructions:

Combine bentonite clay, baking soda, arrowroot powder, and citric acid in a bowl. Mix until you see that there are no more clumps.
In another bowl, combine Castor and Olive Oil together then mix until well combined.
Pour Olive and Castor Oil mixture over the dry ingredients then add Peppermint Essential Oil

and Jellybean Fragrance Oil. Mix until well combined.

Place each of the colorants into separate bowls. Put equal parts of the wet and dry mixture into each of the bowls then mix with your hands until crumbly.

Now, fill up the Easter egg molds with the mixture and leave to dry until 24 hours. Store in mason jars or airtight containers.

Use and enjoy!

Gingerbread Beauty

While you may not be able to eat this bath bomb, you can still indulge in the soothing benefits of ginger because of it! This one is light, soothing, and can also strengthen your respiratory system, as well!

What you'll need:

10 drops Ginger Essential Oil
5 drops Gingersnap Fragrance Oil
1 cup Citric Acid
2 cups Baking Soda
Witch Hazel Spray
40 drops Brown Soap Colorant

Instructions:

In a bowl, mix baking soda and citric acid together then add soap colorant, fragrance oil, and ginger essential oil.

Mix with your hands until crumbly then spray Witch Hazel so there would not be any clumps. Press mixture into the molds then let them dry overnight.

Use and enjoy!

Oh Christmas Tree

And finally, here's a bath bomb that's perfect for the Christmas Season! It's dashed with lemon, too, so it's good for your health!

What you'll need:

Christmas tree Molds
Candy Sprinklers
10 grams Kelly Green Soap Colorant
10 grams Pine Green Soap Colorant
Witch Hazel Spray
10 drops lemon essential oil
28 grams Castor Oil
5 grams Kaolin Clay
8 grams Pine Fragrance Oil
132 grams citric acid
264 grams baking soda

Instructions:

Put the soap colorants in separate bowls and set aside.

In a bowl, mix kaolin clay, baking soda, and citric acid together then in another bowl, mix lemon essential oil, and pine fragrance oil together.

Combine wet and dry ingredients and mix with your hands until crumbly. Spray Witch Hazel for misting.
Put half of the mixture into the pine green bowl and the other in the Kelly green one.

Press into Christmas tree molds then wait for 24 hours so they would be dried.

Once dry, spray Witch Hazel onto each of the molds then press them together and wait overnight to dry.

Use and enjoy!

Conclusion

Thank you for reading this book!

I hope this book was able to help you create fragrant bath bombs that will soothe your soul and improve the state of your help.

Try them out now and indulge in the goodness that they'd bring.

Finally, if you enjoyed this book, please take time to post a review on Amazon. It will be greatly appreciated.

Thank you and enjoy!

Bonus Content

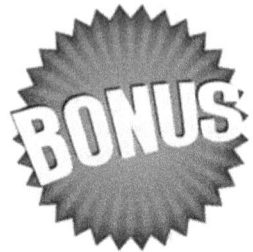

As a token of our appreciation Grand Reveur Publications would like to give you access to our exclusive bonus content (including free eBooks!).

Exclusive pre-release access to our latest eBooks Free Grand Reveur eBooks during promotional periods.

To receive additional bonus content please go to the following web site:

https://ignorelimits.leadpages.net/grandreveur publications/

As this is a limited time offer it would be a shame to miss out, I recommend grabbing these bonuses before reading on